Radiation Therapy and You

A GUIDE TO SELF-HELP DURING TREATMENT

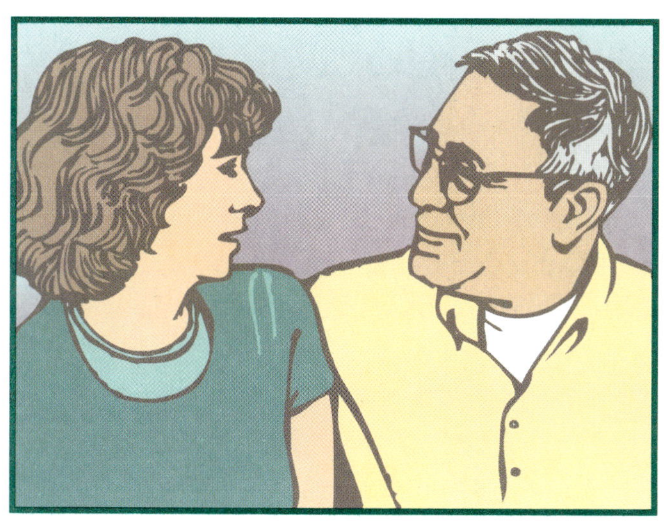

U.S. DEPARTMENT OF HEALTH AND HUMAN SERVICES
Public Health Service
National Institutes of Health

Contents

Acknowledgements

The National Cancer Institute thanks all of the many health professionals and patients who assisted with the development and review of this publication.

Introduction

This booklet is for patients who are receiving radiation therapy for **cancer.** It describes what to expect during therapy and offers suggestions for self-care during and after treatment. It explains the two most common types of radiation therapy: external radiation and internal radiation therapy. Information is included about the general effects of treatment and how to deal with specific side effects.

You may not want to read everything in this booklet at one time. Browse through it, read the sections that are of interest to you right now, and look at the others as needed. Because your doctor will plan the treatment specifically for you and the type of cancer you have, some information may not apply to you.

Radiation therapy may vary somewhat among different doctors, hospitals, and treatment centers. Therefore, your treatment or the advice of your doctor (the radiation oncologist) may be different from what you read here. Be sure to ask questions and discuss your concerns with your doctor, nurse, or radiation therapist. Ask whether they have any additional written information that might help you.

You will find some helpful sections at the back of this booklet:

- The Glossary defines all the words in bold print. Knowing the meanings of words that relate to radiation therapy and cancer treatment can help you understand more about your illness and the roles of the people involved in your treatment.

- The section, "Additional Resources for Cancer Information," tells you how to get more information from the National Cancer Institute about cancer and services for cancer patients.

- The page labeled "Notes" may be used to write down the questions you want to ask your doctor, nurse, or other members of your treatment team.

FAST FACTS ABOUT RADIATION THERAPY

- Radiation treatments are painless.
- External radiation treatment does not make you radioactive.
- Treatments are usually scheduled every day except Saturday and Sunday.
- You need to allow 30 minutes for each treatment session, although the treatment itself takes only a few minutes.
- It's important to get plenty of rest and to eat a well-balanced diet during the course of your radiation therapy.
- Skin in the treated area may become sensitive and easily irritated.
- Side effects of radiation treatment are usually temporary, and they vary depending on the area of the body that is being treated.

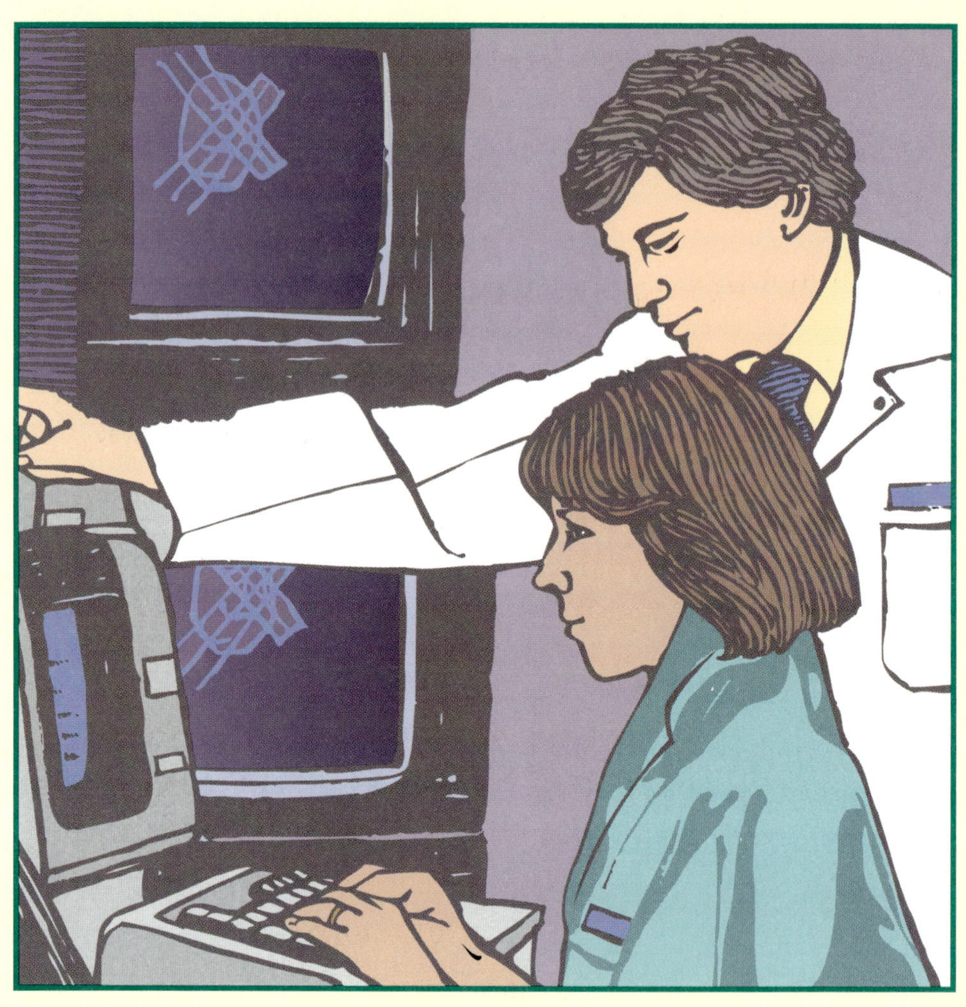

1 Radiation in Cancer Treatment

What Is Radiation Therapy?

Radiation therapy (sometimes called radiotherapy, x-ray therapy, or irradiation) is the treatment of disease using penetrating beams of high energy waves or streams of particles called **radiation.**

Many years ago doctors learned how to use this energy to "see" inside the body and find disease. You've probably seen a chest x-ray or x-ray pictures of your teeth or your bones. At high doses (many times those used for x-ray exams), radiation is used to treat cancer and other illnesses.

The radiation used for cancer treatment comes from special machines or from **radioactive** substances. Radiation therapy equipment aims specific amounts of the radiation at **tumors** or areas of the body where there is disease.

How Does Radiation Therapy Work?

Radiation in high doses kills cells or keeps them from growing and dividing. Because cancer cells grow and divide more rapidly than most of the normal cells around them, radiation therapy can successfully treat many kinds of cancer. Normal cells are also affected by radiation but, unlike cancer cells, most of them recover from the effects of radiation.

To protect normal cells, doctors carefully limit the doses of radiation and spread the treatment out over time. They also shield as much normal tissue as possible while they aim the radiation at the site of the cancer.

What Are the Goals and Benefits of Radiation Therapy?

The goal of radiation therapy is to kill the cancer cells with as little risk as possible to normal cells. Radiation therapy can be used to treat many kinds of cancer in almost any part of the body. In fact, more than half of all people with cancer are treated with some form of radiation. For many cancer patients, radiation is the only kind of treatment they need. Thousands of people who have had radiation therapy alone or in combination with other types of cancer treatment are free of cancer.

Radiation treatment, like surgery, is a local treatment--it affects the cancer cells only in a specific area of the body. Sometimes doctors add radiation therapy to treatments that reach all parts of the body (systemic treatment), such as **chemotherapy**, or **biological therapy**, to improve treatment results. You may hear your doctor use the term **adjuvant therapy** for a treatment that is added to, and given after, the primary therapy.

Radiation therapy is often used with surgery to treat cancer. Doctors may use radiation before surgery to shrink a tumor. This makes it easier to remove the cancerous tissue and may allow the surgeon to perform less radical surgery. Radiation therapy may be used after surgery to stop the growth of cancer cells that may remain. Your doctor may choose to use radiation therapy and surgery at the same time. This procedure, known as **intraoperative radiation,** is explained more fully in this booklet in Chapter 2, "External Radiation Therapy."

In some cases, instead of surgery, doctors use radiation along with anticancer drugs (chemotherapy) to destroy the cancer. Radiation may be given before, during, or after chemotherapy. Doctors carefully tailor this combination treatment to each patient's needs depending on the type of cancer, its location, and its size. The purpose of radiation treatment before or during chemotherapy is to make the tumor smaller and thus improve the effectiveness of the anticancer drugs. Doctors sometimes recommend that a patient complete chemotherapy and then have radiation treatment to kill any cancer cells that might remain.

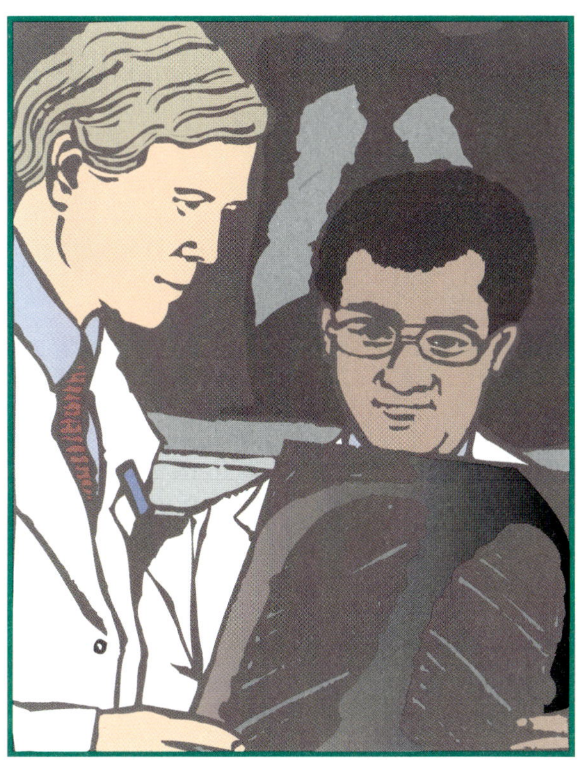

When curing the cancer is not possible, radiation therapy can be used to shrink tumors and reduce pressure, pain, and other symptoms of cancer. This is called **palliative care** or **palliation.** Many cancer patients find that they have a better quality of life when radiation is used for this purpose.

What Are the Risks of Radiation Therapy?

The brief high doses of radiation that damage or destroy cancer cells can also injure or kill normal cells. These effects of radiation on normal cells cause treatment side effects. Most side effects of radiation treatment are well known and, with the help of your doctor and nurse, easily treated. The side effects of radiation therapy and what to do about them are discussed in Chapter 4 of this booklet, "Managing Side Effects."

The risk of side effects is usually less than the benefit of killing cancer cells. Your doctor will not advise you to have any treatment unless the benefits — control of disease and relief from symptoms —are greater than the known risks.

How Is Radiation Therapy Given?

Radiation therapy can be given in one of two ways: external or internal. Some patients have both, one after the other.

Most people who receive radiation therapy for cancer have **external radiation.** It is usually given during outpatient visits to a hospital or treatment center. In external radiation therapy, a machine directs the high-energy rays at the cancer and a small margin of normal tissue surrounding it.

The various machines used for external radiation work in slightly different ways. Some are better for treating cancers near the skin surface; others work best on cancers deeper in the body. The most common type of machine used for radiation therapy is called a **linear accelerator.** Some radiation machines use a variety of radioactive substances (such as cobalt-60, for example) as the source of high-energy rays. Your doctor decides which type of radiation therapy machine is best for you. You will find more information about external radiation in the next chapter.

When **internal radiation** therapy is used, the radiation source is placed inside the body. This method of radiation treatment is called **brachytherapy** or implant therapy. The source of the radiation (such as radioactive iodine, for example) sealed in a small holder is called an **implant.** Implants may be thin wires, plastic tubes (catheters), capsules, or seeds. An implant may be placed directly into a tumor or inserted into a body cavity. Sometimes, after a tumor has been removed by surgery, the implant is placed in the 'tumor bed' (the area from which the tumor was removed) to kill any tumor cells that may remain.

Another type of internal radiation therapy uses unsealed radioactive materials which may be taken by mouth or injected into the body. If you have this type of treatment, you may need to stay in the hospital for several days. More information about internal radiation therapy can be found in Chapter 3.

Who Gives Radiation Treatments?

A doctor who specializes in using radiation to treat cancer — a **radiation oncologist** — will prescribe the type and amount of treatment that is right for you. The radiation oncologist is the person referred to as "your doctor" throughout this booklet. The radiation oncologist works closely with the other doctors and health care professionals involved in your care. This highly trained health care team may include:

- The **radiation physicist**, who makes sure that the equipment is working properly and that the machines deliver the right dose of radiation. The physicist also works closely with your doctor to plan your treatment.
- The **dosimetrist**, who works under the direction of your doctor and the radiation physicist and helps carry out your treatment plan by calculating the amount of radiation to be delivered to the cancer and normal tissues that are nearby.
- The **radiation therapist**, who positions you for your treatments and runs the equipment that delivers the radiation.
- The **radiation nurse**, who will coordinate your care, help you learn about treatment, and tell you how to manage side effects. The nurse can also answer questions you or family members may have about your treatment.

Your health care team also may include a physician assistant, **radiologist**, dietitian, **physical therapist**, social worker, or other health care professional.

Is Radiation Treatment Expensive?

Treatment of cancer with radiation can be costly. It requires very complex equipment and the services of many health care professionals. The exact cost of your radiation therapy will depend on the type and number of treatments you need.

Most health insurance policies, including Part B of Medicare, cover charges for radiation therapy. It's a good idea to talk with your doctor's office staff or the hospital business office about your policy and how expected costs will be paid.

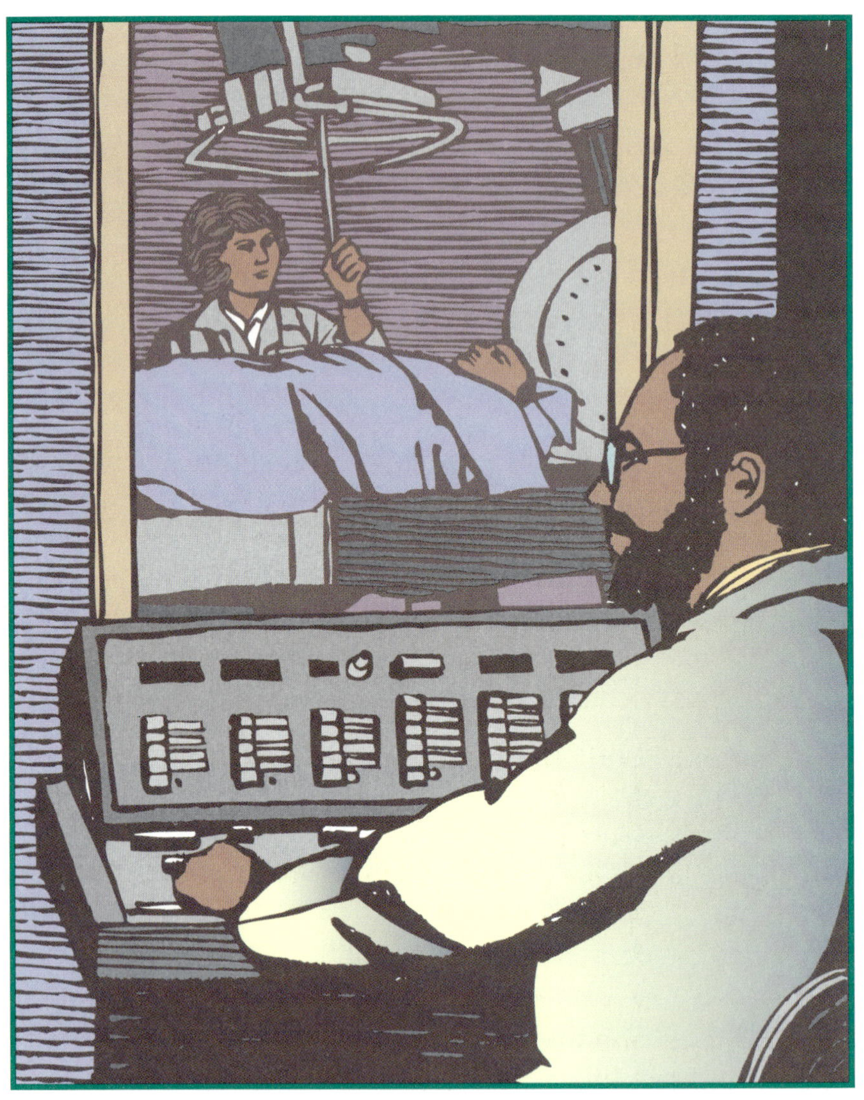

In some states, the Medicaid program may help you pay for treatments. You can find out from the office that handles social services in your city or county whether you are eligible for Medicaid and whether your radiation therapy is a covered expense.

If you need financial aid, contact the hospital social service office or the National Cancer Institute's (NCI) Cancer Information Service at 1-800-4-CANCER. They may be able to direct you to sources of help. Additional sources of cancer information are described in the Resources section at the end of this book.

2 External Radiation Therapy: What To Expect

How Does the Doctor Plan My Treatment?

The high energy rays used for radiation therapy can come from a variety of sources. Your doctor may choose to use **x-rays**, an **electron beam**, or **cobalt-60 gamma rays.** Some cancer treatment centers have special equipment that produces beams of **protons** or **neutrons** for radiation therapy. The type of radiation your doctor decides to use depends on what kind of cancer you have and how far into your body the radiation should go. High-energy radiation is used to treat many types of cancer. Low-energy x-rays are used to treat some kinds of skin diseases.

After a physical exam and a review of your medical history, the doctor plans your treatment. In a process called **simulation**, you will be asked to lie very still on an examining table while the radiation therapist uses a special x-ray machine to define your **treatment port** or **field.** This is the exact place on your body where the radiation will be aimed. Depending on the location of your cancer, you may have more than one treatment port.

Simulation may also involve **CT scans** or other imaging studies to plan how to direct the radiation. Depending on the type of treatment you will be receiving, body molds or other devices that keep you from moving during treatment (immobilization devices) may be made at this time. They will be used each time you have treatment to be sure that you are positioned correctly. Simulation may take from a half-hour to about 2 hours.

The radiation therapist often will mark the treatment port on your skin with tattoos or tiny dots of colored, permanent ink. It's important that the radiation be targeted at the same area each time. If the dots appear to be fading, tell your radiation therapist, who will darken them so that they can be seen easily.

Once simulation has been done, your doctor will meet with the radiation physicist and the dosimetrist. Based on the results of your medical history, lab tests, x-rays, other treatments you may have had, and the location and kind of cancer you have, they will decide how much radiation is needed, what kind of machine to use to deliver it, and how many treatments you should have.

After you have started the treatments, your doctor and the other members of your health care team will follow your progress by checking your response to treatment and how you are feeling at least once a week. When necessary, your doctor may revise the treatment plan by changing the radiation dose or the number and length of your remaining radiation sessions.

Your nurse will be available daily to discuss your concerns and answer any questions you may have. Be sure to tell your nurse if you are having any side effects or if you notice any unusual symptoms.

How Long Does the Treatment Take?

For most types of cancer, radiation therapy is usually given 5 days a week for 6 or 7 weeks. (When radiation is used for palliative care, the course of treatment is shorter, usually 2 to 3 weeks.) The total dose of radiation and the number of treatments you need will depend on the size, location, and kind of cancer you have; your general health; and other medical treatments you may be receiving.

Using many small doses of daily radiation rather than a few large doses helps protect normal body tissues in the treatment area. Weekend rest breaks allow normal cells to recover.

It's very important that you have all of your scheduled treatments to get the most benefit from your therapy. Missing or delaying treatments can lessen the effectiveness of your radiation treatment.

What Happens During the Treatment Visits?

Before each treatment, you may need to change into a hospital gown or robe. It's best to wear clothing that is easy to take off and put on again.

In the treatment room, the radiation therapist will use the marks on your skin to locate the treatment area and to position you correctly. You may sit in a special chair or lie down on a treatment table. For each external radiation therapy session, you will be in the treatment room about 15 to 30 minutes, but you will be getting radiation for only about 1 to 5 minutes of that time. Receiving external radiation treatments is painless, just like having an x-ray taken. You will not hear, see, or smell the radiation.

The radiation therapist may put special shields (or blocks) between the machine and certain parts of your body to help protect normal tissues and organs. There might also be plastic or plaster forms that help you stay in exactly the right place. **You need to remain very still during the treatment so that the radiation reaches only the area where it's needed, and the same area is treated each time.** You don't have to hold your breath — just breathe normally.

The radiation therapist will leave the treatment room before your treatment begins. The radiation machine is controlled from a nearby area. You will be watched on a television screen or through a window in the control room. Although you may feel alone, keep in mind that the therapist can see and hear you and even talk with you using an intercom in the treatment room. If you should feel ill or very uncomfortable during the treatment, tell your therapist at once. The machine can be stopped at any time.

The machines used for radiation treatments are very large, and they make noises as they move around your body to aim at the treatment area from different angles. Their size and motion may be frightening at first. Remember that the machines are being moved and controlled by your radiation therapist. They are checked constantly to be sure they're working right. If you have concerns about anything that happens in the treatment room, discuss these concerns with the radiation therapist.

What Is Hyperfractionated Radiation Therapy?

Radiation is usually given once daily in a dose that is based on the type and location of the tumor. In **hyperfractionated radiation** therapy, the daily dose is divided into smaller doses that are given more than once a day. The treatments usually are separated by 4 to 6 hours. Doctors are studying hyperfractionated therapy to learn if it is equal to, or perhaps more effective than, once-a-day therapy and whether there are fewer long-term side effects. Early results of treatment studies of some kinds of tumors are encouraging, and hyperfractionated therapy is becoming a more common way to give radiation treatments for some types of cancer.

What Is Intraoperative Radiation?

Intraoperative radiation combines surgery and radiation therapy. The surgeon first removes as much of the tumor as possible. Before the surgery is completed, a large dose of radiation is given directly to the tumor bed (the area from which the tumor has been removed) and nearby areas where cancer cells might have spread. Sometimes intraoperative radiation is used in addition to external radiation therapy. This gives the cancer cells a larger amount of radiation than would be possible using external radiation alone.

IMPROVING RADIATION TREATMENT

Researchers in the field of radiation therapy continue to seek ways to improve the outcome of treatment. Their challenge is to get a high dose of radiation to the tumor while the surrounding normal tissue is protected from radiation damage. New methods for using radiation to treat cancer are being investigated. Many are promising, but they are not yet widely available. You may hear the following terms that describe some of these new methods of radiation treatment:

Three-dimensional conformal radiation therapy is a radiation technique that is being used in some cancer centers. Computer simulation produces an accurate image of the tumor and surrounding organs so that multiple radiation beams can be shaped exactly to the contour of the treatment area. Because the radiation beams are precisely focused, nearby normal tissue is spared. This technique is being used to treat prostate cancer, lung cancer, and certain brain tumors.

Stereotactic radiosurgery, which uses gamma rays or a linear accelerator, is useful for treating certain kinds of brain tumors and some malformations in the brain's blood vessels. One technique, called the "**gamma knife,**" uses many powerful, precisely focused radiation beams. The patient wears a special helmet to focus the gamma rays and aim them at the target tissue from many directions. The treatment is painless and bloodless and, unlike conventional brain surgery, there is no danger of infection. Other systems use a linear accelerator to deliver the radiation in arcing paths around the patient's head.

The **cyberknife** is a new, but less common, treatment that is being used to treat brain tumors. This system uses a miniature radiation machine and a robotic arm that moves around the patient's head while delivering small doses of radiation from hundreds of directions. During treatment, a computer analyzes hundreds of brain images and adjusts for slight movements by the patient. This makes it possible to deliver the treatment without using a frame to hold the patient's head still. Only the tumor receives the high doses of radiation, and healthy tissue is spared.

The **Peacock system** is a variation of the cyberknife. It uses special machinery that delivers tiny focused beams of radiation while it rotates around the patient's head. The beams continuously change shape and size to conform to the shape and size of the tumor while avoiding vital structures in the brain. Computer software controls the intensity of the radiation.

Precision therapy is a method of radiosurgery recently developed in Sweden. It uses high doses of radiation delivered in fewer fractions than in conventional radiation therapy. An advanced treatment planning system permits precise targeting from many angles. As with other advances in radiation treatment, it allows high doses of radiation to be delivered to tumor tissue while reducing radiation damage to healthy tissue.

What Are the Side Effects of Treatment?

External radiation therapy does not cause your body to become radioactive. There is no need to avoid being with other people because you are undergoing treatment. Even hugging, kissing, or having sexual relations with others poses no risk of radiation exposure.

Most side effects of radiation therapy are related to the area that is being treated. Many patients have no side effects at all. Your doctor and nurse will tell you about the possible side effects you might expect and how you should deal with them. You should contact your doctor or nurse if you have any unusual symptoms during your treatment, such as coughing, sweating, fever, or pain.

The side effects of radiation therapy, although unpleasant, are usually not serious and can be controlled with medication or diet. They usually go away within a few weeks after treatment ends, although some side effects can last longer. In Chapter 4, "Managing Side Effects," you will find advice on how to cope with the side effects that might occur during and after your therapy. Always check with your doctor or nurse about how you should deal with side effects.

Throughout your treatment, your doctor will regularly check on the effects of the treatment. You may not be aware of changes in the cancer, but you probably will notice decreases in pain, bleeding, or other discomfort. You may continue to notice further improvement after your treatment is completed.

Your doctor may recommend periodic tests and physical exams to be sure that the radiation is causing as little damage to normal cells as possible. Depending on the area being treated, you may have routine blood tests to check the levels of **red blood cells, white blood cells**, and **platelets**; radiation treatment can cause decreases in the levels of different blood cells.

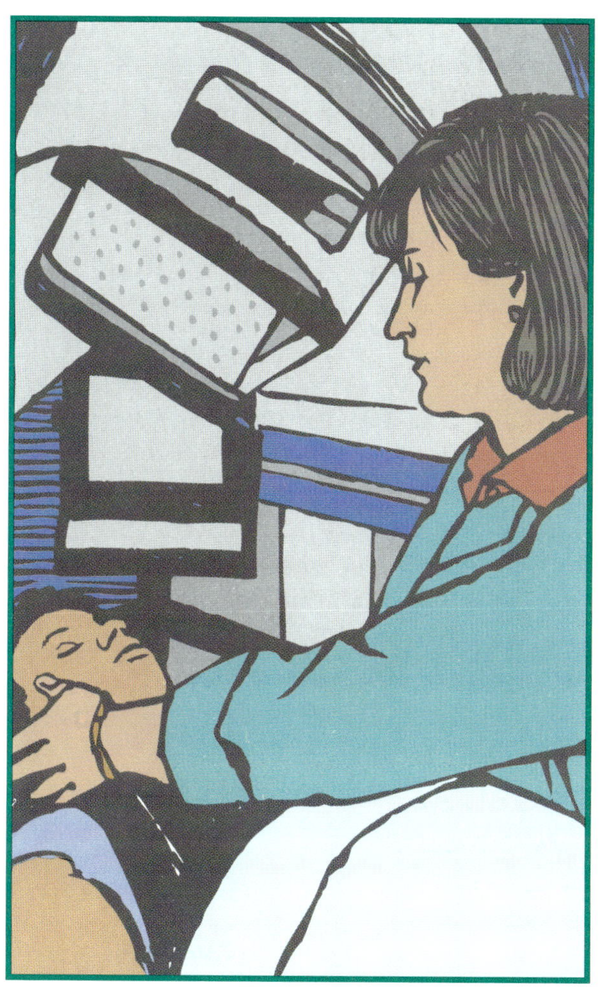

What Can I Do To Take Care of Myself During Therapy?

Each patient's body responds to radiation therapy in its own way. That's why your doctor must plan, and sometimes adjust, your treatment. In addition, your doctor or nurse will give you suggestions for caring for yourself at home that are specific to your treatment and the possible side effects.

Nearly all cancer patients receiving radiation therapy need to take special care of themselves to protect their health and to help the treatment succeed. Some guidelines to remember are given on the following pages:

- **Before starting treatment, be sure your doctor knows about any medicines you are taking and if you have any allergies.** Do not start taking any medicine (whether prescription or over-the-counter) during your radiation therapy without first telling your doctor or nurse.

- **Fatigue is common during radiation therapy.** Your body will use a lot of extra energy over the course of your treatment, and you may feel very tired. Be sure to get plenty of rest, and sleep as often as you feel the need. It's common for fatigue to last for 4 to 6 weeks after your treatment has been completed.

- **Good nutrition is very important.** Try to eat a balanced diet that will prevent weight loss. For patients who have problems with eating or diet planning, the chapter, "Managing Side Effects," offers practical tips.

- **Check with your doctor before taking vitamin supplements or herbal preparations during treatment.**

- **Avoid wearing tight clothes, such as girdles or close-fitting collars, over the treatment area.**

- **Be extra kind to your skin in the treatment area:**
  - Ask your doctor or nurse if you may use soaps, lotions, deodorants, sun blocks, medicines, perfumes, cosmetics, talcum powder, or other substances in the treated area.
  - Wear loose, soft cotton clothing over the treated area.
  - Do not wear starched or stiff clothing over the treated area.
  - Do not scratch, rub, or scrub treated skin.

- Do not use adhesive tape on treated skin. If bandaging is necessary, use paper tape and apply it outside of the treatment area. Your nurse can help you place dressings so that you can avoid irritating the treated area.
- Do not apply heat or cold (heating pad, ice pack, etc.) to the treated area. Use only lukewarm water for bathing the area.
- Use an electric shaver if you must shave the treated area but only after checking with your doctor or nurse. Do not use a preshave lotion or hair removal products on the treated area.
- Protect the treatment area from the sun. Do not apply sunscreens just before a radiation treatment. If possible, cover treated skin with light clothing before going outside. Ask your doctor if you should use a sunscreen or a sun-blocking product. If so, select one with a protection factor of at least 15 and reapply it often. Ask your doctor or nurse how long after your treatments are completed you should continue to protect the treated skin from sunlight.

■ **If you have questions, ask your doctor or nurse.** They are the only ones who can properly advise you about your treatment, its side effects, home care, and any other medical concerns you may have.

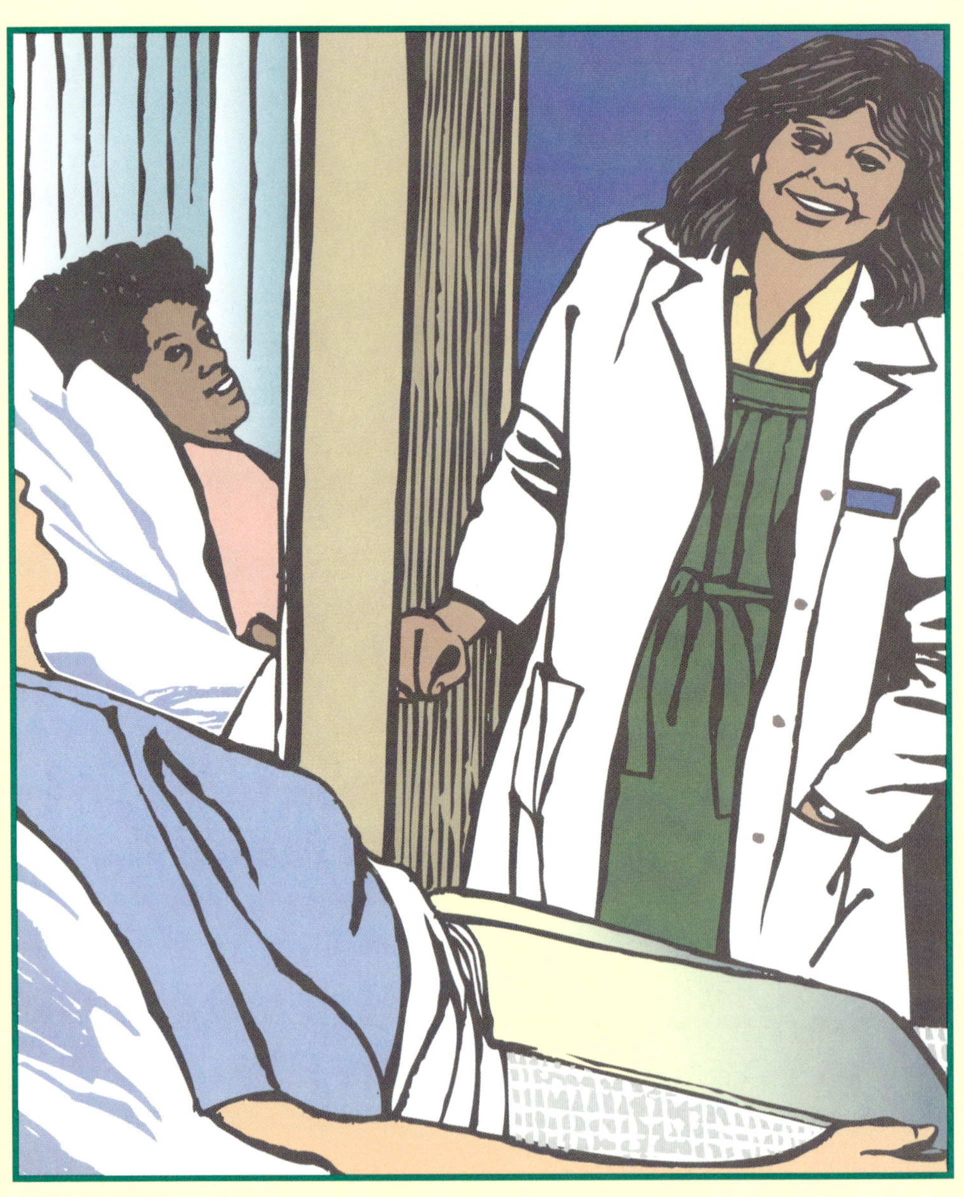

3 Internal Radiation Therapy: What To Expect

When Is Internal Radiation Therapy Used?

Your doctor may decide that a high dose of radiation given to a small area of your body is the best way to treat your cancer. Internal radiation therapy allows the doctor to give a higher total dose of radiation in a shorter time than is possible with external treatment.

Internal radiation therapy places the radiation source as close as possible to the cancer cells. Instead of using a large radiation machine, the radioactive material, sealed in a thin wire, catheter, or tube (implant), is placed directly into the affected tissue. This method of treatment concentrates the radiation on the cancer cells and lessens radiation damage to some of the normal tissue near the cancer. Some of the radioactive substances used for internal radiation treatment include cesium, iridium, iodine, phosphorus, and palladium.

Internal radiation therapy may be used for cancers of the head and neck, breast, uterus, thyroid, cervix, and prostate. Your doctor may suggest using both internal and external radiation therapy.

In this booklet, "internal radiation treatment" refers to implant radiation. Health professionals prefer to use the term "brachytherapy" for implant radiation therapy. You may hear your doctor or nurse use the terms, **interstitial radiation** or **intracavitary radiation**; each is a form of internal radiation therapy. Sometimes radioactive implants are called "capsules" or "seeds."

How Is the Implant Placed in the Body?

The type of implant and the method of placing it depend on the size and location of the cancer. Implants may be put right into the tumor (interstitial radiation), in special applicators inside a body cavity (intracavitary radiation) or passage (intraluminal radiation), on the surface of a tumor, or in the area from which the tumor has been removed. Implants may be removed after a short time or left in place permanently. If they are to be left in place, the radioactive substance used will lose radiation quickly and become nonradioactive in a short time.

When interstitial radiation is given, the radiation source is placed in the tumor in **catheters**, seeds, or capsules. When intracavitary radiation is used, a container or applicator of radioactive material is placed in a body cavity such as the uterus. In surface brachytherapy, the radioactive source is sealed in a small holder and placed in or against the tumor. In intraluminal brachytherapy the radioactive source is placed in a body **lumen** or tube, such as the bronchus or esophagus.

Internal radiation also may be given by injecting a solution of radioactive substance into the bloodstream or a body cavity. This form of radiation therapy may be called **unsealed internal radiation therapy.**

For most types of implants, you will need to be in the hospital. You will be given general or local **anesthesia** so that you will not feel any pain when the doctor places the holder for the radioactive material in your body. In many hospitals, the radioactive material is placed in its holder or applicator after you return to your room so that other patients, staff, and visitors are not exposed to radiation.

How Are Other People Protected From Radiation While the Implant is in Place?

Sometimes the radiation source in your implant sends its high energy rays outside your body. To protect others while you are having implant therapy, the hospital will have you stay in a private room. Although the nurses and other people caring for you

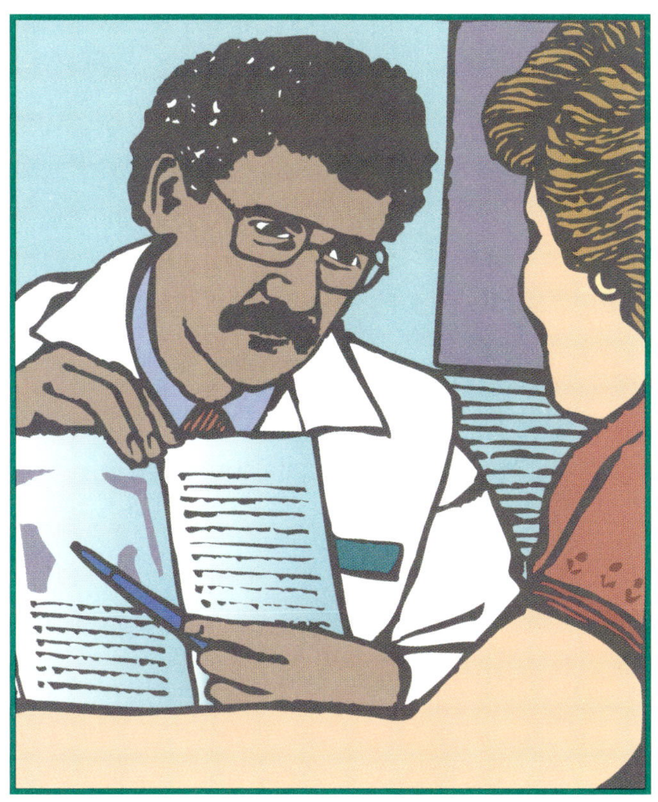

will not be able to spend a long time in your room, they will give you all of the care you need. You should call for a nurse when you need one, but keep in mind that the nurse will work quickly and speak to you from the doorway more often than at your bedside. In most cases, your urine and stool will contain no radioactivity unless you are having unsealed internal radiation therapy.

There also will be limits on visitors while your implant is in place. Children younger than 18 and pregnant women should not visit patients who are having internal radiation therapy. Be sure to tell your visitors to ask the hospital staff for any special instructions before they come into your room. Visitors should sit at least 6 feet from your bed, and the radiation oncology staff will determine how long your visitors may stay. The time can vary from 30 minutes to several hours per day. In some hospitals, a rolling lead shield is placed beside the bed and kept between the patient and visitors or staff members.

What Are the Side Effects of Internal Radiation Therapy?

The side effects of implant therapy depend on the area being treated. You are not likely to have severe pain or feel ill during implant therapy. However, if an applicator is holding your implant in place, it may be somewhat uncomfortable. If you need it, the doctor will order medicine to help you relax or to relieve pain. If general anesthesia was used while your implant was put in place, you may feel drowsy, weak, or nauseated, but these effects do not last long. If necessary, medications can be ordered to relieve nausea.

Be sure to tell the nurse about any symptoms that concern you. In Chapter 4, "Managing Side Effects," you will find tips on how to deal with problems that might occur after implant therapy.

How Long Does the Implant Stay in Place?

Your doctor will decide the amount of time that an implant is to be left in place. It depends on the dose (amount) of radioactivity needed for effective treatment. Your treatment schedule will depend on the type of cancer, where it is located, your general health, and other cancer treatments you have had. Depending on where the implant is placed, you may have to keep it from shifting by staying in bed and lying fairly still.

Temporary implants may be either low dose-rate (LDR) or high dose-rate (HDR). Low dose-rate implants are left in place for several days; high dose-rate implants are removed after a few minutes.

For some cancer sites, the implant is left in place permanently. If your implant is permanent, you may need to stay in your hospital room away from other people for a few days while the radiation is most active. The implant becomes less radioactive each day; by the time you are ready to go home, the radiation in your body will be much weaker. Your doctor will advise you if there are any special precautions you need to take at home.

What Happens After the Implant Is Removed?

Usually, an anesthetic is not needed when the doctor removes a temporary implant. Most can be taken out right in the patient's hospital room. Once the implant is removed, there is no radioactivity in your body. The hospital staff and your visitors will no longer have to limit the time they stay with you.

Your doctor will tell you if you need to limit your activities after you leave the hospital. Most patients are allowed to do as much as they feel like doing. You may need some extra sleep or rest breaks during your days at home, but you should feel stronger quickly.

The area that has been treated with an implant may be sore or sensitive for some time. If any particular activity, such as sports or sexual intercourse, causes irritation in the treatment area, your doctor may suggest that you limit this activity for a while.

REMOTE BRACHYTHERAPY

In **remote brachytherapy,** a computer sends the radioactive source through a tube to a catheter that has been placed near the tumor by the patient's doctor. The procedure is directed by the brachytherapy team, who watch the patient on closed-circuit television and communicate with the patient using an intercom. The radioactivity remains at the tumor for only a few minutes. In some cases, several remote treatments may be required, and the catheter may stay in place between treatments.

Remote brachytherapy may be used for low dose-rate (LDR) treatments in an inpatient setting. **High dose-rate (HDR) remote brachytherapy** allows a person to have internal radiation therapy in an outpatient setting. High dose-rate treatments take only a few minutes. Because no radioactive material is left in the body, the patient can return home after the treatment. Remote brachytherapy has been used to treat cancers of the cervix, breast, lung, pancreas, prostate, and esophagus.

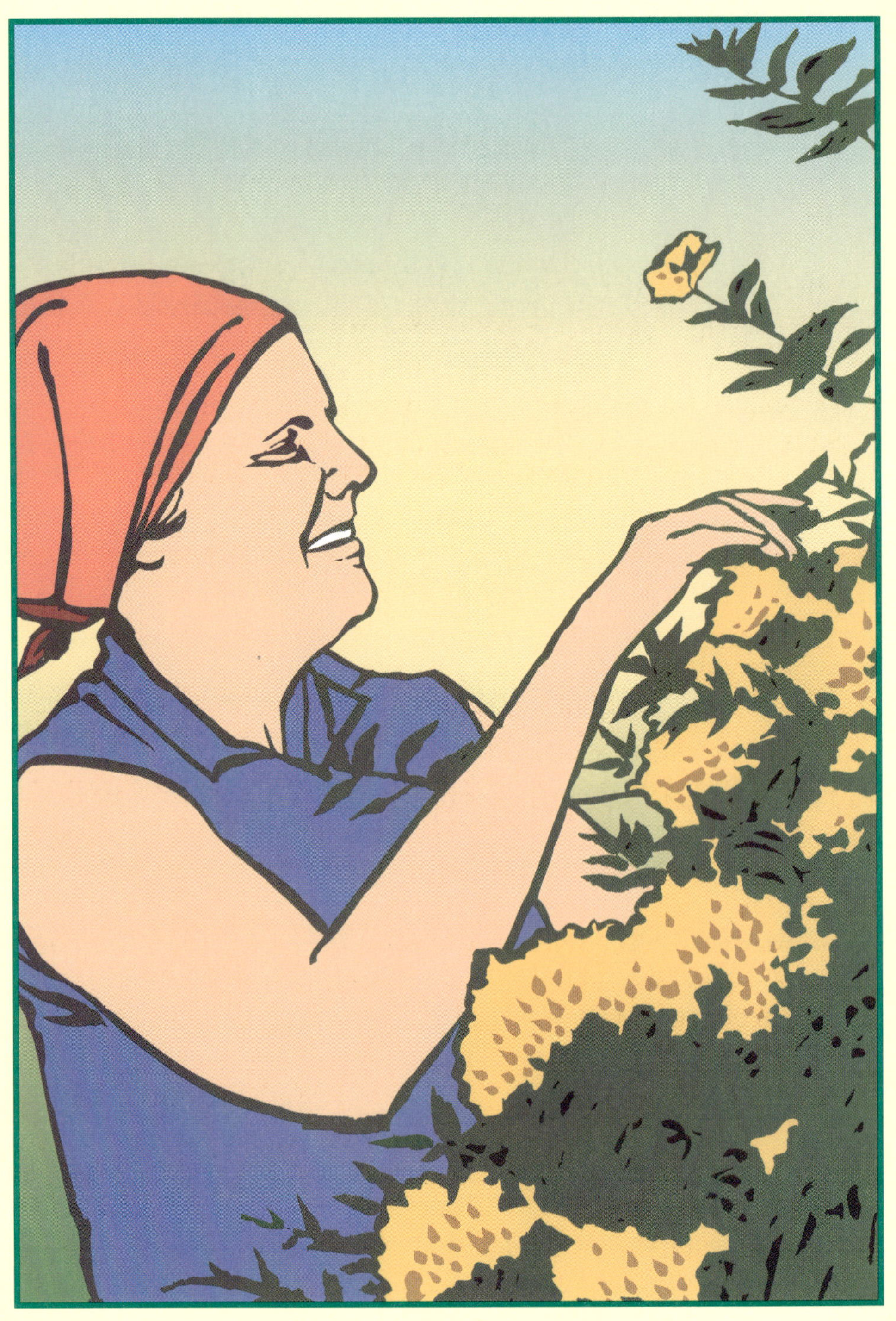

4 *Managing Side Effects*

Are Side Effects the Same for Everyone?

The side effects of radiation treatment vary from patient to patient. You may have no side effects or only a few mild ones through your course of treatment. Some people do experience serious side effects, however. The side effects that you have depend mostly on the radiation dose and the part of your body that is treated. Your general health also can affect how your body reacts to radiation therapy and whether you have side effects. Before beginning your treatment, your doctor and nurse will discuss the side effects you might experience, how long they might last, and how serious they might be.

Side effects may be acute or chronic. Acute side effects are sometimes referred to as "early side effects." They occur soon after the treatment begins and usually are gone within a few weeks of finishing therapy. Chronic side effects, sometimes called "late side effects," may take months or years to develop and usually are permanent.

The most common early side effects of radiation therapy are fatigue and skin changes. They can result from radiation to any treatment site. Other side effects are related to treatment of specific areas. For example, temporary or permanent hair loss may be a side effect of radiation treatment to the head. Appetite can be altered if treatment affects the mouth, stomach, or intestine. This chapter discusses common side effects first. Then the side effects that involve specific areas of the body are described.

Fortunately, most side effects will go away in time. In the meantime, there are ways to reduce discomfort. If you have a side effect that is especially severe, the doctor may prescribe a break in your treatments or change your treatment in some way.

Be sure to tell your doctor, nurse, or radiation therapist about any side effects that you notice. They can help you treat the problems and tell you how to lessen the chances that the side effects will come back. The information in this booklet can serve as a guide to handling some side effects, but it cannot take the place of talking with the members of your health care team.

Will Side Effects Limit My Activity?

Not necessarily. It will depend on which side effects you have and how severe they are. Many patients are able to work, prepare meals, and enjoy their usual leisure activities while they are having radiation therapy. Others find that they need more rest than usual and therefore cannot do as much. Try to continue doing the things you enjoy as long as you don't become too tired.

Your doctor may suggest that you limit activities that might irritate the area being treated. In most cases, you can have sexual relations if you wish. You may find that your desire for physical intimacy is lower because radiation therapy may cause you to feel more tired than usual. For most patients, these feelings are temporary. (See "Sexual Relations" later in this chapter.)

What Causes Fatigue?

Fatigue, feeling tired and lacking energy, is the most common symptom reported by cancer patients. The exact cause is not always known. It may be due to the disease itself or to treatment. It may also result from lowered blood counts, lack of sleep, pain, and poor appetite.

Most people begin to feel tired after a few weeks of radiation therapy. During radiation therapy, the body uses a lot of energy for healing. You also may be tired because of stress related to your illness, daily trips for treatment, and the effects of radiation on normal cells. Feelings of weakness or weariness will go away gradually after your treatment has been completed.

You can help yourself during radiation therapy by not trying to do too much. If you do feel tired, limit your activities and use your leisure time in a restful way. Save your energy for doing the

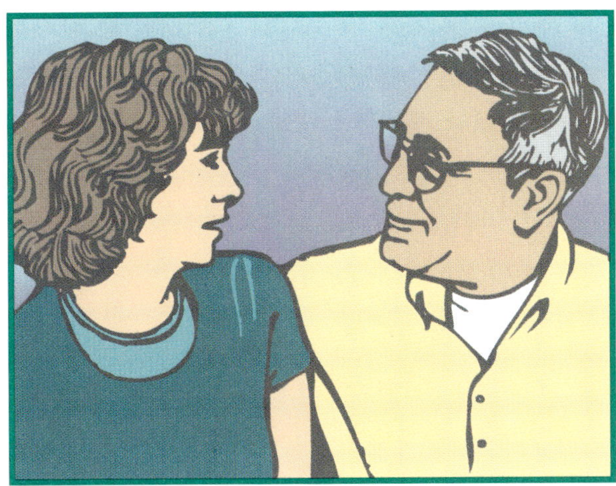

things that you feel are most important. Do not feel that you have to do everything you normally do. Try to get more sleep at night, and plan your day so that you have time to rest if you need it. Several short naps or breaks may be more helpful than a long rest period.

Sometimes, light exercise such as walking may combat fatigue. Talk with your doctor or nurse about how much exercise you may do while you are having therapy. Talking with other cancer patients in a support group may also help you learn how to deal with fatigue.

If you have a full-time job, you may want to try to continue to work your normal schedule. However, some patients prefer to take time off while they're receiving radiation therapy; others work a reduced number of hours. Speak frankly with your employer about your needs and wishes during this time. A part-time schedule may be possible, or perhaps you can do some work at home. Ask your doctor's office or the radiation therapy department to help by trying to schedule treatments with your workday in mind.

Whether you're going to work or not, it's a good idea to ask family members or friends to help with daily chores, shopping, childcare, housework, or driving. Neighbors may be able to help by picking up groceries for you when they do their own shopping. You also could ask someone to drive you to and from your treatment visits to help conserve your energy.

How Are Skin Problems Treated?

You may notice that your skin in the treatment area is red or irritated. It may look as if it is sunburned or tanned. After a few weeks, your skin may be very dry from the therapy. Ask your doctor or nurse for advice on how to relieve itching or discomfort.

With some kinds of radiation therapy, treated skin may develop a "moist reaction," especially in areas where there are skin folds. When this happens, the skin is wet, and it may become very sore. It's important to notify your doctor or nurse if your skin develops a moist reaction. They can give you suggestions on how to care for these areas and prevent them from becoming infected. Other tips on skin care can be found in the chapter on external radiation therapy.

During radiation therapy, you will need to be very gentle with the skin in the treatment area. The following suggestions may be helpful:

- Avoid irritating treated skin.
- When you wash, use only lukewarm water and mild soap; pat dry.
- Do not wear tight clothing over the area.
- Do not rub, scrub, or scratch the skin in the treatment area.
- Avoid putting anything that is hot or cold, such as heating pads or ice packs, on your treated skin.
- Ask your doctor or nurse to recommend skin care products that will not cause skin irritation. Do not use any powders, creams, perfumes, deodorants, body oils, ointments, lotions, or home remedies in the treatment area while you're being treated, and for several weeks afterward, unless approved by your doctor or nurse.
- Do not apply any skin lotions within 2 hours of a treatment.

- Avoid exposing the radiated area to the sun during treatment. If you expect to be in the sun for more than a few minutes, you will need to be very careful. Wear protective clothing (such as a hat with a broad brim and a shirt with long sleeves) and use a sunscreen. Ask your doctor or nurse about using sunblocking lotions. After your treatment is over, ask your doctor or nurse how long you should continue to take extra precautions in the sun.

The majority of skin reactions to radiation therapy go away a few weeks after treatment is completed. In some cases, though, the treated skin will remain slightly darker than it was before and it may continue to be more sensitive to sun exposure.

What Can Be Done About Hair Loss?

Radiation therapy can cause hair loss, also known as **alopecia**, but only in the area being treated. For example, if you are receiving treatment to your hip, you will not lose the hair from your head. Radiation of your head may cause you to lose some or all of the hair on your scalp. Many patients find that their hair grows back again after the treatments are finished. The amount of hair that grows back will depend on how much and what kind of radiation you receive. You may notice that your hair has a slightly different texture or color when it grows back. Other types of cancer treatment, such as chemotherapy, can also affect how your hair grows back.

Although your scalp may be tender after the hair is lost, it's a good idea to cover your head with a hat, turban, or scarf. You should wear a protective cap or scarf when you're in the sun or outdoors in cold weather. If you prefer a wig or toupee, be sure the lining does not irritate your scalp. The cost of a hairpiece that you need because of cancer treatment is a tax-deductible expense and may be covered in part by your health insurance. If you plan to buy a wig, it's a good idea to select it early in your treatment if you want to match the color and style to your own hair.

How are Side Effects on the Blood Managed?

Radiation therapy can cause low levels of white blood cells and platelets. These blood cells normally help your body fight infection and prevent bleeding. If large areas of active bone marrow are treated, your red blood cell count may be low as well. If your blood tests show these side effects, your doctor may wait to continue treatments until your blood counts increase. Your doctor will check your blood counts regularly and change your treatment schedule if it is necessary.

Will Eating Be a Problem?

Sometimes radiation treatment causes loss of appetite and interferes with eating, digesting, and absorbing food. Try to eat enough to help damaged tissues rebuild themselves. It is not unusual to lose 1 or 2 pounds a week during radiation therapy. You will be weighed weekly to monitor your weight.

It is very important to eat a balanced diet. You may find it helpful to eat small meals often and to try to eat a variety of different foods. Your doctor or nurse can tell you whether you should eat a special diet, and a **dietitian** will have some ideas that will help you maintain your weight.

Coping with short-term diet problems may be easier than you expect. There are a number of diet guides and recipe booklets for patients who need help with eating problems. A National Cancer Institute booklet, **Eating Hints for Cancer Patients** explains how to get more calories and protein without eating more food. It also has many tips that should help you enjoy eating. The recipes it contains can be used for the whole family and are marked for people with special concerns such as low-salt diets. (To obtain this booklet, see the section at the end of this book, "Additional Resources for Cancer Information.")

If it's painful to chew and swallow, your doctor may advise you to use a powdered or liquid diet supplement. Many of these products are available at drugstores and supermarkets and come in a variety of flavors. They are tasty when used alone or combined with other foods, such as pureed fruit, or added to milkshakes.

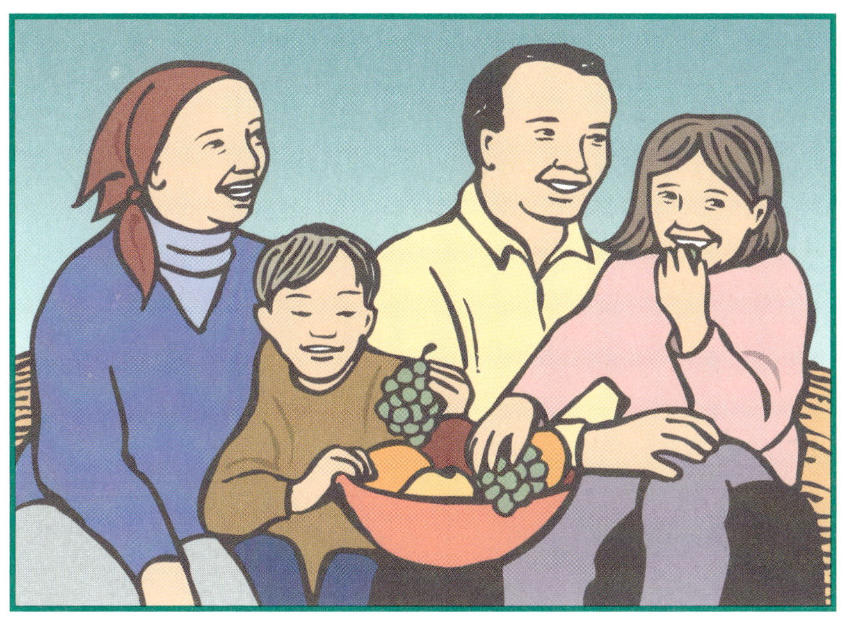

Some of the companies that make these diet supplements have recipe booklets to help you increase your nutrient intake. Ask your nurse, dietitian, or pharmacist for further information.

You may lose interest in food during your treatment. Fatigue from your treatments can cause loss of appetite. Some people just don't feel like eating because of stress from their illness and treatment or because the treatment changes the way food tastes. Even if you're not very hungry, it's important to keep your protein and calorie intake high. Doctors have found that patients who eat well can better cope with having cancer and with the side effects of treatment. Medications for appetite enhancement are now available; ask your doctor or nurse about them.

The list below suggests ways to perk up your appetite when it's poor and to make the most of it when you do feel like eating.

- Eat when you are hungry, even if it is not mealtime.
- Eat several small meals during the day rather than three large ones.
- Use soft lighting, quiet music, brightly colored table settings, or whatever helps you feel good while eating.

- Vary your diet and try new recipes. If you enjoy company while eating, try to have meals with family or friends. It may be helpful to have the radio or television on while you eat.

- Ask your doctor or nurse whether you can have a glass of wine or beer with your meal to increase your appetite. Keep in mind that, in some cases, alcohol may not be allowed because it could worsen the side effects of treatment. This may be especially true if you are receiving radiation therapy for cancer of the head, neck, or upper chest area, including the esophagus.

- Keep simple meals in the freezer to use when you feel hungry.

- If other people offer to cook for you, let them. Don't be shy about telling them what you'd like to eat.

- Keep healthy snacks close by for nibbling when you get the urge.

- If you live alone, you might want to arrange for "Meals on Wheels" to bring food to you. Ask your doctor, nurse, social worker, or local social service agencies about "Meals on Wheels." This service is available in most large communities.

If you are able to eat only small amounts of food, you can increase the calories per serving by:

- Adding butter or margarine.

- Mixing canned cream soups with milk or half-and-half rather than water.

- Drinking eggnog, milkshakes, or prepared liquid supplements between meals.

- Adding cream sauce or melted cheese to your favorite vegetables.

Some people find they can drink large amounts of liquids even when they don't feel like eating solid foods. If this is the case for you, try to get the most from each glassful by making drinks enriched with powdered milk, yogurt, honey, or prepared liquid supplements.

Will Radiation Therapy Affect Me Emotionally?

Nearly all patients being treated for cancer report feeling emotionally upset at different times during their therapy. It's not unusual to feel anxious, depressed, afraid, angry, frustrated, alone, or helpless. Radiation therapy may affect your emotions indirectly through fatigue or changes in hormone balance, but the treatment itself is not a direct cause of mental distress.

You may find that it's helpful to talk about your feelings with a close friend, family member, chaplain, nurse, social worker, or psychologist with whom you feel at ease. You may want to ask your doctor or nurse about meditation or relaxation exercises that might help you unwind and feel calmer.

Nationwide support programs can help cancer patients to meet others who share common problems and concerns. Some medical centers have formed peer support groups so that patients can meet to discuss their feelings and inspire each other.

There are several helpful books, tapes, and videos on dealing with the emotional effects of having cancer. You may find that the National Cancer Institute publication, **Taking Time**, is a good resource for this kind of information. (To obtain this booklet, see the section at the back of this book, "Additional Resources for Cancer Information.")

The Cancer Information Service (1-800-4-CANCER) can direct you to reading matter and other resources in your area for emotional support.

What Side Effects Occur With Radiation Therapy to the Head and Neck?

Some people who receive radiation to the head and neck experience redness, irritation, and sores in the mouth; a dry mouth or thickened saliva; difficulty in swallowing; changes in taste; or nausea. Try not to let these symptoms keep you from eating.

Other problems that may occur during treatment to the head and neck are a loss of taste, which may diminish appetite and affect nutrition, and earaches (caused by hardening of ear wax).

You may notice some swelling or drooping of the skin under your chin as well as changes in the skin texture. Your jaw may also feel stiff and you may be unable to open your mouth as wide as before treatment. Jaw exercises may help ease this problem. Report all side effects to your doctor or nurse and ask what you should do about them.

If you are receiving radiation therapy to the head or neck, you need to take especially good care of your teeth, gums, mouth, and throat. Side effects from treatment to these areas commonly involve the mouth, which may be sore and dry.

Here are a few tips that may help you manage mouth problems:

- Avoid spices and coarse foods such as raw vegetables, dry crackers, and nuts.
- Remember that acidic foods and liquids can cause mouth and throat irritation.
- Don't smoke, chew tobacco, or drink alcohol.
- Stay away from sugary snacks, because they can promote tooth decay.
- Clean your mouth and teeth often, using the method your dentist or doctor recommends.
- Use only alcohol-free mouthwash; many commercial mouth-washes contain alcohol, which has a drying effect on mouth tissues.

MOUTH CARE

Radiation treatment for head and neck cancer can increase your chances of getting cavities in your teeth. Mouth care designed to prevent problems will be a very important part of your treatment. Before starting radiation therapy, make an appointment for a complete dental/oral checkup. Ask your dentist and radiation oncologist to consult before your radiation treatments begin.

Your dentist probably will want to see you often during your radiation therapy to help you care for your mouth and teeth. This is a good way to reduce the risk of tooth decay and help you deal with possible problems, such as soreness of the tissues in your mouth. It's important that you follow the dentist's advice while you're receiving radiation therapy. Most likely, your dentist will suggest that you:

- Clean your teeth and gums thoroughly with a soft brush at least 4 times a day (after meals and at bedtime).
- Use a **fluoride** toothpaste that contains no abrasives.
- Floss gently between teeth daily if you flossed regularly before your illness. Use waxed, non-shredding dental floss.
- Rinse your mouth gently and frequently with a salt and baking soda solution, especially after you brush. Use 1/2 teaspoon of salt and 1/2 teaspoon of baking soda in a large glass of warm water. Follow with a plain water rinse.
- Apply fluoride regularly as prescribed by your dentist.

Your dentist can explain how to mix the salt and baking soda mouthwash and how to use the fluoride treatment method that best suits your needs. You can probably get printed instructions for proper dental care at the dentist's office. If dry mouth continues after your treatment is complete, you will need to continue the mouth care recommended during treatment. Always share your dentist's instructions with your radiation nurse.

DEALING WITH MOUTH OR THROAT PROBLEMS

Soreness in your mouth or throat may appear in the second or third week of external radiation therapy, and it will most likely have disappeared within a month or so after your treatments have ended. You may have trouble swallowing during this time because your mouth feels dry. Your doctor or dentist can prescribe medicine for mouth discomfort and tell you about methods to relieve other mouth problems during and following your radiation therapy. If you wear dentures, you may notice that they no longer fit well. This occurs if the radiation causes your gums to swell. You may need to stop wearing your dentures until your radiation therapy is over. It's important not to risk denture-induced gum sores, because they may become infected and heal slowly.

Your salivary glands may produce less saliva than usual, making your mouth feel dry. Unfortunately, dry mouth may continue to be a problem even after treatment is over. You may be given medication to help lessen this side effect. It's helpful to sip cool drinks throughout the day. Although many radiation therapy patients have said that drinking carbonated beverages helps relieve dry mouth, water is probably your best choice. In the morning, fill a large container with ice, add water, and carry it with you during the day so that you can take frequent sips. Keep a glass of cool water at your bedside at night, too. Sugar-free candy or gum also may help; be careful about overuse of these products as they can cause diarrhea in some people. Avoid tobacco and alcoholic drinks because they tend to dry and irritate your mouth tissues. Moisten food with gravies and sauces to make eating easier. If these measures are not enough, ask your dentist, radiation oncologist, or nurse about products that either replace or stimulate your own saliva. Artificial saliva and medication to increase saliva production are available.

TIPS ON EATING

You may find that it's difficult or painful to swallow. Some patients say that they feel as if something is stuck in their throats. Soreness or dryness in your mouth or throat can also make it hard to eat. The earlier section in this booklet on eating problems may be helpful. In addition, some of the following tips may help to make eating more comfortable:

- Choose foods that taste good to you and are easy to eat.
- Try changing the consistency of foods by adding fluids and using sauces and gravies to make them softer.
- Avoid highly spiced foods and foods with textures that are dry and rough, such as crackers.
- Eat small meals, and eat more frequently than usual.
- Cut your food into small, bite-sized pieces.
- Ask your doctor for special liquid medicines to reduce the pain in your throat so that you can eat and swallow more easily.

- Ask your doctor about liquid food supplements that are easier to swallow than solids. They can help you get enough calories each day to avoid losing weight.
- If you are being treated for lung cancer, it's important to keep mucus and other secretions thin and manageable; drinking extra fluids can help.
- If familiar foods no longer taste good, try new foods and use different methods of food preparation.

Additional helpful suggestions can be found in the NCI booklet, **Eating Hints for Cancer Patients.**

What Side Effects Occur With Radiation Therapy to the Chest?

Radiation treatment to the chest may cause several changes. For example, you may find that it is hard to swallow or that swallowing hurts. You may develop a cough or a fever. You may notice that when you cough the amount and color of the mucus is different. Shortness of breath is also common. Be sure to let your treatment team know right away if you have any of these symptoms. Remember that your doctor and nurse have seen these changes in many radiation patients, and they know how to help you deal with them.

Are There Side Effects With Radiation Therapy for Breast Cancer?

The most common side effects with radiation therapy for breast cancer are fatigue and skin changes. However, there may be other side effects as well. If you notice that your shoulder feels stiff, ask your doctor or nurse about exercises to keep your arm moving freely. Other side effects include breast or nipple soreness, swelling from fluid buildup in the treated area, and skin reddening or tanning. Except for tanning, which may take up to 6 months to fade, these side effects will most likely disappear in 4 to 6 weeks.

If you are being treated for breast cancer and you are having radiation therapy after a lumpectomy or mastectomy, it's a good idea to go without your bra whenever possible or, if this makes you more uncomfortable, wear a soft cotton bra without underwires. This will help reduce skin irritation in the treatment area.

Radiation therapy after a lumpectomy may cause additional changes in the treated breast after therapy is complete. These long-term side effects may continue for a year or longer after treatment. The skin redness will fade, leaving your skin slightly darker, just as when a sunburn fades to a suntan. The pores in the skin of your breast may be enlarged and more noticeable. Some women report increased sensitivity of the skin on the breast; others have decreased feeling. The skin and the fatty tissue of the breast may feel thicker and firmer than they were before your radiation treatment. Sometimes, the size of your breast changes — it may become larger because of fluid buildup or smaller because of the development of scar tissue. Many women have little or no change in size.

Your radiation therapy plan may include temporary implants of radioactive material in the area around your lumpectomy. A week or two after external treatment is completed, these implants are inserted during a short hospitalization. The implants may cause breast tenderness or a feeling of tightness. After they are removed, you are likely to notice some of the same effects that occur with external treatment. If so, let your doctor or nurse know about any problems that persist.

Most changes resulting from radiation therapy for breast cancer are seen within 10 to 12 months after completing therapy. Occasionally small red areas called **telangiectasias** appear. These are areas of dilated blood vessels, and the color may fade with time. If you see new changes in breast size, shape, appearance, or texture after this time, report them to your doctor at once.

What Side Effects Occur With Radiation Therapy to the Stomach and Abdomen?

If you are having radiation treatment to the stomach or some portion of the abdomen, you may have an upset stomach, nausea, or diarrhea. Your doctor can prescribe medicines to relieve these problems. Do not take any medications for these symptoms unless you first check with your doctor or nurse.

MANAGING NAUSEA

It's not unusual to feel queasy for a few hours right after radiation treatment to the stomach or abdomen. Some patients find that they have less nausea if they have their treatment on an empty stomach. Others report that eating a light meal 1 to 2 hours before treatment lessens queasiness. You may find that nausea is less of a problem if you wait 1 to 2 hours after your treatment before you eat. If this problem persists, ask your doctor to prescribe a medicine (an **antiemetic**) to prevent nausea. If antiemetics are prescribed, take them within the hour before treatment or when your doctor or nurse suggests, even if you sometimes feel that they are not needed.

If your stomach feels upset just before every treatment, the queasiness or nausea may be caused by anxiety and concerns about cancer treatment. Try having a bland snack such as toast or crackers and apple juice before your appointment. It may also help to try to unwind before your treatment. Reading a book, writing a letter, or working a crossword puzzle may help you relax.

Here are some other tips to help an unsettled stomach:

- Stick to any special diet that your doctor, nurse, or dietitian gives you.
- Eat small meals.
- Eat often and try to eat and drink slowly.
- Avoid foods that are fried or are high in fat.
- Drink cool liquids between meals.
- Eat foods that have only a mild aroma and can be served cool or at room temperature.

For severe nausea and vomiting, try a clear liquid diet (broth and clear juices) or bland foods that are easy to digest, such as dry toast and gelatin.

WHAT TO DO ABOUT DIARRHEA

Diarrhea may begin in the third or fourth week of radiation therapy to the abdomen or pelvis. You may be able to prevent diarrhea by eating a low fiber diet when you start therapy: avoid foods such as raw fruits and vegetables, beans, cabbage, and wholegrain breads and cereals. Your doctor or nurse may suggest other changes to your diet, prescribe antidiarrhea medicine, or give you special instructions to help with the problem. Tell the doctor or nurse if these changes fail to control your diarrhea. The following changes in your diet may help:

- Try a clear liquid diet (water, weak tea, apple juice, clear broth, plain gelatin) as soon as diarrhea starts or when you feel that it's going to start.
- Ask your doctor or nurse to advise you about liquids that won't make your diarrhea worse. Weak tea and clear broth are frequent suggestions.
- Avoid foods that are high in fiber or can cause cramps or a gassy feeling, such as raw fruits and vegetables, coffee and other beverages that contain caffeine, beans, cabbage, wholegrain breads and cereals, sweets, and spicy foods.
- Eat frequent, small meals.
- If milk and milk products irritate your digestive system, avoid them or use lactose-free dairy products.
- Continue a diet that is low in fat and fiber and lactose-free for 2 weeks after you have finished your radiation therapy. Gradually reintroduce other foods. You may want to start with small amounts of low-fiber foods such as rice, bananas, applesauce, mashed potatoes, low-fat cottage cheese, and dry toast.
- Be sure your diet includes foods that are high in potassium (bananas, potatoes, apricots), an important mineral that you may lose through diarrhea.

Diet planning is very important for patients who are having radiation treatment of the stomach and abdomen. Try to pack the highest possible food value into every meal and snack so that you will be eating enough calories and vital nutrients. Remember that nausea, vomiting, and diarrhea are likely to disappear once your treatment is over.

What Side Effects Occur With Radiation Therapy to the Pelvis?

If you are having radiation therapy to any part of the pelvis (the area between your hips), you might have some of the digestive problems already described. You also may have bladder irritation, which can cause discomfort or frequent urination. Drinking a lot of fluid can help relieve some of this discomfort. Avoid caffeine and carbonated beverages. Your doctor also can prescribe some medicine to help relieve these problems.

The effects of radiation therapy on sexual and reproductive functions depend on which organs are in the radiation treatment area. Some of the more common side effects do not last long after treatment is finished. Others may be long-term or permanent. Before your treatment begins, ask your doctor about possible side effects and how long they might last.

Depending on the radiation dose, women having radiation therapy in the pelvic area may stop menstruating and have other symptoms of menopause such as vaginal itching, burning, and dryness. You should report these symptoms to your doctor or nurse, who can suggest treatment.

EFFECTS ON FERTILITY

Scientists are still studying how radiation treatment affects fertility. If you are a woman in your childbearing years, it's important to discuss birth control and fertility issues with your doctor. You should not become pregnant during radiation therapy because radiation treatment during pregnancy may injure the fetus, especially in the first 3 months. If you are pregnant before your therapy begins, be sure to tell your doctor so that the fetus can be protected from radiation, if possible.

Radiation therapy to the area that includes the testes can reduce both the number of sperm and their effectiveness. This does not mean that conception cannot occur, however. Ask your doctor or nurse about effective measures to prevent pregnancy while you are having radiation. If you have any concerns about fertility, be sure to discuss them with your doctor. For example, if you want to have children, you may be concerned about reduced fertility after your cancer treatment is completed. Your doctor can help you get information about the option of banking your sperm before treatment.

SEXUAL RELATIONS

With most types of radiation therapy, neither men nor women are likely to notice any change in their ability to enjoy sex. Both sexes, however, may notice a decrease in their level of desire. This is more likely to be due to the stress of having cancer than to the effects of radiation therapy. Once the treatment ends, sexual desire is likely to return to previous levels.

During radiation treatment to the pelvis, some women are advised not to have intercourse. Others may find that intercourse is uncomfortable or painful. Within a few weeks after treatment ends, these symptoms usually disappear. If shrinking of vaginal tissues occurs as a side effect of radiation therapy, your doctor or nurse can explain how to use a dilator, a device that gently stretches the tissues of the vagina.

If you have questions or concerns about sexual activity during and after cancer treatment, discuss them with your nurse or doctor. Ask them to recommend booklets that may be helpful.

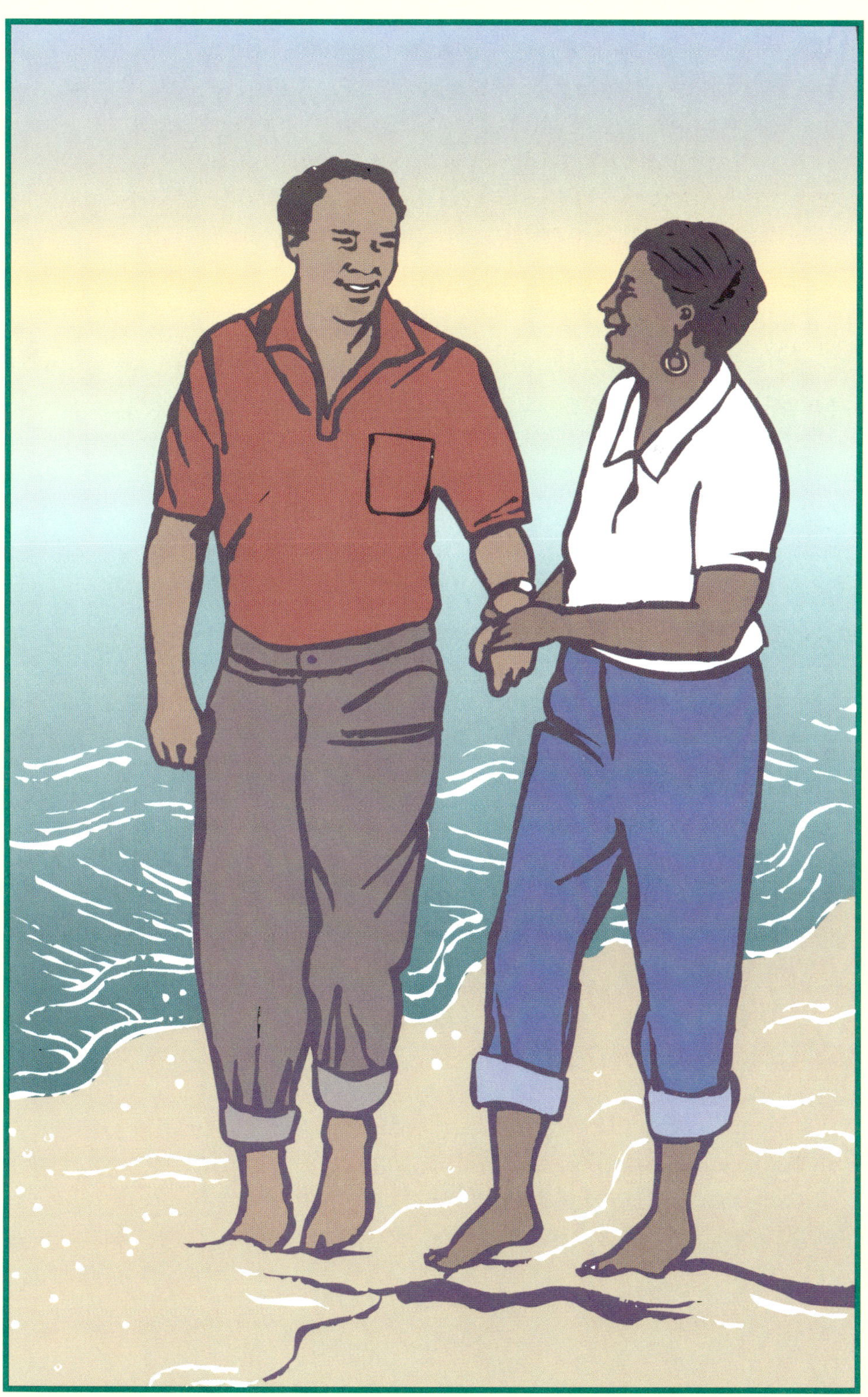

5 Followup Care

What Does "Followup" Mean?

Once you have completed your radiation treatments, it is important for your doctor to monitor the results of your therapy at regularly scheduled visits. These checkups are necessary to deal with radiation side effects and to detect any signs of **recurrent** disease. During these checkups, your doctor will examine you and may order some lab tests and x-rays. The radiation oncologist also will want to see you for followup after your treatment ends and will coordinate followup care with your doctor.

Followup care might include more cancer treatment, rehabilitation, and counseling. Taking good care of yourself is also an important part of following through after radiation treatments.

Who Provides Care After Therapy?

Most patients return to the radiation oncologist for regular followup visits. Others are referred to their original doctor, to a surgeon, or to a **medical oncologist.** Your followup care will depend on the kind of cancer that was treated and on other treatments that you had or may need.

What Other Care Might Be Needed?

Just as every patient is different, followup care varies. Your doctor will prescribe and schedule the followup care that you need. Don't hesitate to ask about the tests or treatments that your doctor orders. Try to learn all the things you need to do to take good care of yourself.

Following are some questions that you may want to ask your doctor after you have finished your radiation therapy:

- How often do I need to return for checkups?
- Why do I need more x-rays, CT scans, blood tests, and so on? What will these tests tell us?
- Will I need chemotherapy, surgery, or other treatments?
- How and when will you know if I'm cured of cancer?
- What are the chances that it will come back?
- How soon can I go back to my regular activities? Work? Sexual activity? Sports?
- Do I need to take any special precautions like staying out of the sun or avoiding people with infectious diseases?
- Do I need a special diet?
- Should I exercise?
- Can I wear a **prosthesis**?
- Can I have **reconstructive surgery**? How soon can I schedule it?

It's a good idea to write down the questions you want to ask your doctor. Use the "Notes" page at the back of this booklet for your questions and take it with you when you have your appointment with the doctor. Some patients find that it's helpful to take a family member with them to help remember what the doctor says.

What if Pain Is a Problem?

Radiation therapy is not painful. However, some radiation side effects may cause discomfort. In addition, when radiation is used for palliation (see page 9), some discomfort or pain may remain. Sometimes patients need help to manage cancer pain. Over-the-counter pain medicine may be enough for mild pain. Remember that you should not use a heating pad or a warm compress to relieve pain in any area treated with radiation.

If your pain is severe, ask the doctor about prescription drugs or other methods of relief. Try to be specific about your pain (How severe is it on a scale of 0-10, where 0 is no pain and 10 is the worst pain you can imagine? Where is your pain? Is the pain throbbing, stabbing, searing? Is it continuous or intermittent? What makes it better or worse?) when you tell the doctor about it so you can get the best pain management. If you are unable to get pain relief, you may want to ask your doctor for a referral to a pain specialist.

Because fear and worry can make pain worse, you may find that relaxation exercises are helpful. Other methods, such as hypnosis, biofeedback, and acupuncture, may be useful for some cancer pain. Be sure to discuss these complementary or alternative treatments with your doctor or nurse. Sometimes complementary therapies can interfere with other treatment you are having. They can also be harmful when combined with other treatment.

Questions and Answers About Pain Control: A Guide for People with Cancer and Their Families is a free booklet that may help you understand more about controlling cancer pain. (To obtain this booklet, see "Additional Resources for Cancer Information" at the back of this book.)

How Can I Help Myself After Radiation Therapy?

Patients who have had radiation therapy need to continue some of the special care they used during treatment, at least for a short while. For instance, you may have skin problems for several weeks after your treatments end. Continue to be gentle with skin in the treatment area until all signs of irritation are gone. Don't try to scrub off the marks in your treatment area. If tattoos were used to mark the treatment area, they are permanent and will not wash off. Your nurse can answer questions about skin care and help you with other concerns you may have after your treatment has been completed.

You may find that you still need extra rest after your therapy is over, while your healthy tissues are recovering and rebuilding. Keep taking naps as needed, and try to get more sleep at night. It may take some time to get your strength back, so resume your normal schedule of activities gradually. If you feel that you need emotional or social support, ask your doctor, nurse, or a social worker for information about support groups or other ways to express your feelings and concerns.

When Should I Call the Doctor?

After treatment for cancer, you're likely to be more aware of your body and to notice even slight changes in how you feel from day to day. The doctor will want to know if you are having any unusual symptoms. Promptly tell your doctor about:

- A pain that doesn't go away, especially if it's always in the same place.
- New or unusual lumps, bumps, or swelling.
- Nausea, vomiting, diarrhea, or loss of appetite.
- Unexplained weight loss.
- A fever or cough that doesn't go away.
- Unusual rashes, bruises, or bleeding.
- Any symptoms that you are concerned about.
- Any other warning signs mentioned by your doctor or nurse.

What About Returning to Work?

Many people find that they can continue to work during radiation therapy because treatment appointments are short. If you have stopped working, you can return to your job as soon as you feel up to it. If your job requires lifting or heavy physical activity, you may need a change in your work responsibilities until you have regained your strength. Check with your employer to see if a "Return to Work" release from your doctor is required.

When you are ready to return to work, it is important to learn about your rights regarding your job and health insurance. If you have any questions about employment issues, contact the Cancer Information Service (CIS). CIS staff can help you find local agencies that can help you deal with problems regarding employment and insurance rights that are sometimes faced by cancer survivors.

Conclusion

We hope that the information in this booklet will help you understand how radiation therapy is used to treat cancer. If you know what to expect when you go for your treatments, you may not feel as anxious. Remember to talk with your nurse, doctor, or other members of your health care team whenever you have questions or feel that you need more information.

Glossary

These are the words that appear in bold print in *Radiation Therapy and You.* You also may hear members of your health team use them. Don't be afraid to ask your health care staff to explain any terms you don't understand.

Adjuvant therapy: Treatment added to the primary treatment to enhance the effectiveness of the primary treatment. Radiation therapy often is used as an adjuvant to surgery.

Alopecia *(al-oh-PEE-she-ah)*: Hair loss.

Anesthesia: Loss of feeling or sensation to prevent pain. Certain drugs or gases called 'anesthetics' are used to achieve anesthesia so that medical procedures may be performed without pain. A local anesthetic causes loss of feeling in part of the body. A general anesthetic puts the patient to sleep.

Antiemetic *(an-tee-eh-MET-ik)*: A medicine that prevents or relieves nausea and vomiting.

Biological therapy: Treatment to stimulate or restore the ability of the immune system to fight infection and disease; also called immunotherapy.

Brachytherapy *(BRAK-ee-THER-ah-pee)*: Internal radiation therapy using an implant of radioactive material placed directly into or near the tumor; also called "internal radiation therapy."

Cancer: A term for diseases in which abnormal cells divide without control. Cancer cells can invade nearby tissues and can spread through the bloodstream and lymphatic system to other parts of the body.

Catheter: A thin, flexible, hollow tube through which fluids enter or leave the body. Radioactive materials may be placed in catheters that are placed near the cancer.

Chemotherapy: Treatment with anticancer drugs.

Cobalt 60: A radioactive substance used as a radiation source to treat cancer.

CT (computerized tomography) scan: An x-ray procedure that uses a computer to produce a series of detailed pictures of a cross-section of the body; also called a CAT scan.

Dietitian (also "registered dietitian"): A professional who plans diet programs for proper nutrition.

Dosimetrist *(do-SIM-uh-trist)*: A person who plans and calculates the proper radiation dose for treatment.

Electron beam: A stream of electrons (small, negatively charged particles found in atoms) that can be used for radiation therapy.

External radiation: The use of radiation from a machine located outside of the body to aim high-energy rays at cancer cells.

Fluoride: A chemical applied to the teeth to prevent tooth decay.

Gamma knife: Radiation therapy in which high energy rays are aimed at a brain tumor from many angles in a single treatment session.

Gamma rays: High-energy rays that come from a radioactive source such as cobalt-60.

High dose-rate remote brachytherapy: A type of internal radiation treatment in which the radioactive source is removed between treatments; also known as 'high dose-rate remote radiation therapy.'

Hyperfractionated radiation: Radiation treatment that is given in smaller-than-usual doses two or three times a day.

Implant: A radioactive source in a small holder that is placed in the body in or near a cancer.

Internal radiation: Radiation therapy that uses the technique of placing a radioactive source in or near a cancer.

Interstitial radiation: A radioactive source (implant) placed directly into the cancerous tissue, such as in the head and neck region or the breast.

Intracavitary radiation: A radioactive source (implant) placed in a body cavity, such as the chest cavity or the vagina.

Intraoperative radiation: External radiation treatment given during surgery to deliver a large dose of radiation to the tumor bed and surrounding tissue; also called IORT.

Linear accelerator: A machine that creates high-energy radiation to treat cancers, using electricity to form a stream of fast-moving subatomic particles; also called "mega-voltage (MeV) linear accelerator" or a "linac."

Lumen: The cavity or channel within a tube or tubular organ such as a blood vessel or the intestine.

Medical oncologist: A doctor who specializes in treating cancer with chemotherapy.

Neutron: A small, uncharged particle of matter found in the atoms of all elements except hydrogen. Streams of neutrons generated by special equipment can be used for radiation treatment.

Oncologist: A doctor who specializes in treating cancer.

Palliative care, palliation: Treatment that relieves symptoms but does not cure disease. Palliative care can help people with cancer live more comfortably.

Physical therapist: A health professional trained in the use of such treatments as exercise and massage.

Platelets: Blood cells that help stop bleeding by contributing to the formation of clots.

Prosthesis: An artificial replacement for a body part.

Proton: A small, positively charged particle of matter found in the atoms of all elements. Streams of protons generated by special equipment can be used for radiation treatment.

Radiation: Energy carried by waves or a stream of particles.

Radiation nurse: A nurse who specializes in caring for people who are undergoing radiation therapy.

Radiation oncologist: A doctor who specializes in treating cancer with radiation.

Radiation physicist: The person who makes sure that the radiation machine delivers the right amount of radiation to the treatment site. In consultation with the radiation oncologist, the physicist also determines the treatment schedule that will have the best chance of killing the most cancer cells.

Radiation therapist: The person who runs the equipment that delivers the radiation.

Radiation therapy: Treatment with high-energy rays (such as x-rays) to kill cancer cells. The radiation may come from outside of the body (external radiation) or from radioactive materials placed directly in the tumor (internal or implant radiation). Types of radiation include x-rays, electron beams, gamma rays, neutron beams, and proton beams. Radioactive substances include cobalt, iridium, and cesium. (See also **gamma rays, brachytherapy,** and **x-ray.**)

Radioactive: Capable of emitting high-energy rays or particles.

Radiologist: A doctor with special training in creating and interpreting pictures of areas inside the body. The pictures are produced with x-rays, sound waves, or other types of energy.

Reconstructive surgery: Surgical procedure done to restore the shape of an area of the body altered by cancer surgery.

Recurrence: Reappearance of cancer cells at the same site or in another location after a disease-free period.

Red blood cells: Cells that carry oxygen to all parts of the body. Also called "erythrocytes."

Remote brachytherapy: See **high dose-rate remote brachytherapy.**

Simulation: The process used to plan radiation therapy so that the target area is precisely located and marked.

Telangiectasia: A skin lesion that results from dilation of a group of small blood vessels.

Treatment port or **treatment field:** The place on the body at which the radiation beam is aimed.

Tumor: An abnormal mass of excess tissue that results from excessive cell division. Tumors perform no useful body function and may be either benign (not cancerous) or malignant (cancerous).

Unsealed internal radiation therapy: Internal radiation therapy given by injecting a radioactive substance into the bloodstream or a body cavity. This substance is not sealed in a container.

White blood cells: Cells that help the body fight infection and disease.

X-rays: High-energy radiation that is used in low doses to diagnose disease and in high doses to treat cancer.

Additional Resources for Cancer Information

You may want more information for yourself, your family, and your doctor. The following National Cancer Institute (NCI) services are available to help you.

Telephone...

CANCER INFORMATION SERVICE (CIS)

Provides accurate, up-to-date information on cancer to patients and their families, health professionals, and the general public. Information specialists translate the latest scientific information into understandable language and respond in English, Spanish, or on TTY equipment.

Toll-free: 1-800-4-CANCER (1-800-422-6237)

TTY: 1-800-332-8615

Internet...

These Web sites may be useful:

http://cancer.gov

NCI's primary Web site. Contains information about the Institute and its programs.

http://cancertrials.nci.nih.gov

cancerTrials. NCI's comprehensive clinical trials information center for patients, health professionals, and the public.

Includes information on understanding trials, deciding whether to participate in trials, and finding specific trials, plus research news and other resources.

http://cancernet.nci.nih.gov

CancerNet™. Contains material for health professionals, patients, and the public, including information from PDQ® about cancer treatment, screening, prevention, supportive care, genetics, and clinical trials, and CANCERLIT®, a bibliographic database.

E-mail...

CANCERMAIL

Includes NCI information about cancer treatment, screening, prevention, and supportive care. To obtain a contents list, send e-mail to cancermail@icicc.nci.nih.gov, with the word "help" in the body of the message.

Fax...

CANCERFAX®

CancerFax® includes NCI information about cancer treatment, screening, prevention, and supportive care. To obtain a contents list, dial 301-402-5874 from a fax machine handset and follow the recorded instructions.

Publications...

Cancer patients, their families and friends, and others may find the following National Cancer Institute books useful. They are available free of charge by calling 1-800-4-CANCER.

- *Chemotherapy and You: A Guide to Self-Help During Treatment*
- *Eating Hints for Cancer Patients Before, During, and After Treatment*
- *Get Relief From Cancer Pain*
- *Helping Yourself During Chemotherapy*
- *Questions and Answers About Pain Control: A Guide for People with Cancer and Their Families*
- *Taking Time: Support for People With Cancer and the People Who Care About Them*
- *Taking Part in Clinical Trials: What Cancer Patients Need to Know*

PUBLICATIONS AVAILABLE IN SPANISH...

- *Datos sobre el tratamiento de quimioterapia contra el cancer*
- *El tratamiento de radioterapia; guia para el paciente durante el tratamiento*
- *En que consisten los estudios clinicos? Un folleto para los pacientes de cancer*

Video...

Taking Part in Cancer Clinical Trials: Patient to Patient

Notes

Take this page with you when you go for treatment or when you see your doctor.

Radiation Oncologist

Name ______________________________

Telephone ____________________

Radiation Nurse

Name ______________________________

Telephone ____________________

Other Hospital Contact

Name ______________________________

Telephone ____________________

Transportation

Name ______________________________

Telephone ____________________

Appointments

Date	Time	Location

Questions to Ask